MW01102069

The Library of Sexual Health™

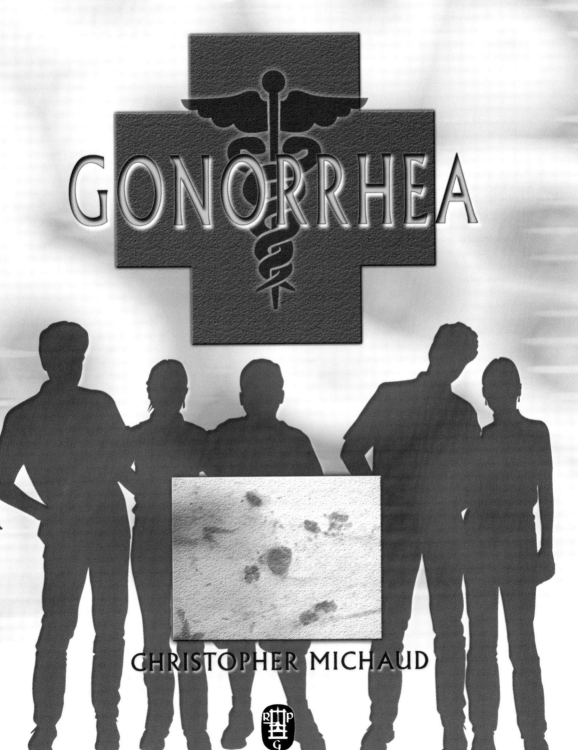

GONORRHEA

CHRISTOPHER MICHAUD

The Rosen Publishing Group, Inc., New York

Published in 2007 by The Rosen Publishing Group, Inc.
29 East 21st Street, New York, NY 10010

Copyright © 2007 by The Rosen Publishing Group, Inc.

First Edition

All rights reserved. No part of this book may be reproduced in any form without permission in writing from the publisher, except by a reviewer.

Library of Congress Cataloging-in-Publication Data

Michaud, Christopher.
Gonorrhea/Christopher Michaud.
    p. cm.—(The library of sexual health)
ISBN-13: 978-1-4042-0908-4
ISBN-10: 1-4042-0908-5 (library binding)
1. Gonorrhea—Juvenile literature. I. Title. II. Series.
RC202.M56 2006
616.95'15—dc22

2006006384

Manufactured in the United States of America

CONTENTS

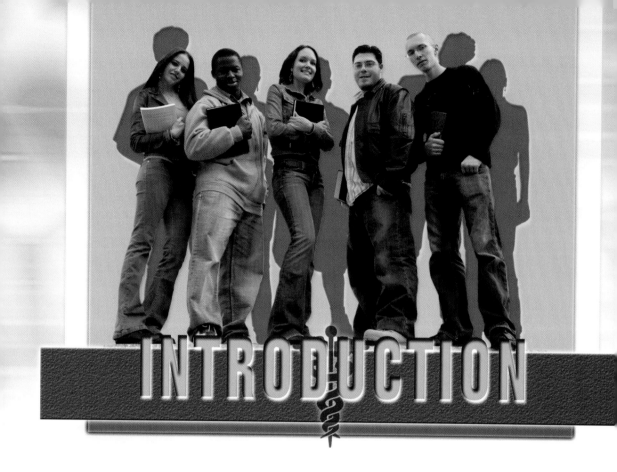

INTRODUCTION

B eing a teenager can be exciting, and sometimes a little scary. Everything seems to be changing all at once. Your body is growing in different ways, you're developing new kinds of relationships with people, you might be starting to date, and you may be experiencing brand-new emotions. With all of these things happening to you and your friends, there are a lot of things you need to learn.

One of the most significant issues involves your health. As you get older, it's important to be well informed about how to make decisions to keep yourself safe and well. Your sexual health is involved in this, too. Learning

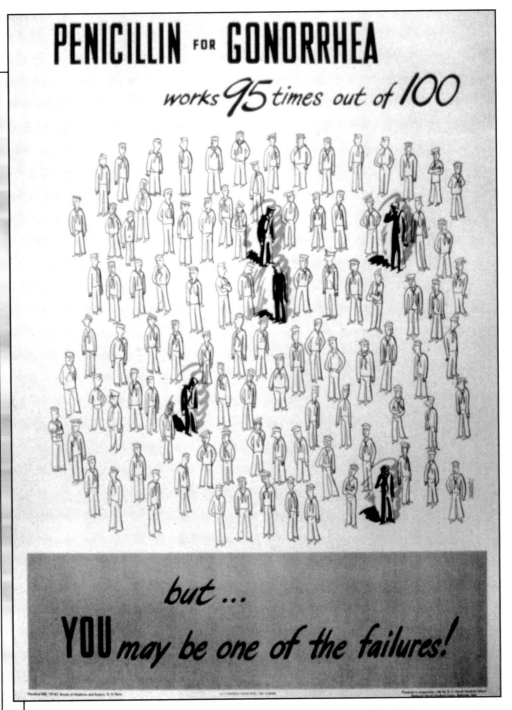

This poster from the World War II era is an example of how the U.S. government tried to educate people about gonorrhea at that time (1941–1945).

about what risks and responsibilities are involved in a sexual relationship is a big part of growing up.

One of these responsibilities is learning how to protect yourself and your partner from sexually transmitted diseases (STDs). An STD is a kind of disease that you can get from having sexual contact with another person. All STDs can be treated, and some can be cured. They can be serious, however, and sometimes even fatal. Sexually transmitted diseases affect people all over the world. Millions of people, including young people, are infected with STDs every year. Fortunately, by being smart and making good choices, the spread of STDs can be prevented. One of the most important tools for this is information. By communicating with other people, like family members, your teachers, the people you date, and your sexual partners, you can take responsibility for your own health and well-being.

This book provides information about gonorrhea, one of the most common, and oldest, sexually transmitted diseases. It explains what gonorrhea is, how you can get it, how a doctor is able to tell if you have it, and how it can be treated. This book also helps you learn how to protect yourself from contracting gonorrhea, or any other STD, in the first place. Lists of further resources at the end of the book can be used to gain more information. Education is one of the best tools we have to prevent the spread of sexually transmitted diseases like gonorrhea.

CHAPTER ONE

About Gonorrhea

Gonorrhea is a common and highly contagious STD. It is one of the world's oldest-known diseases. Hippocrates, a Greek physician, wrote about patients with symptoms of gonorrhea as long ago as 500 BC. Even the word "gonorrhea" has existed for centuries. In the year AD 130, a doctor named Galen came up with the word, which is Greek for "flow of seed." (Galen mistakenly thought that the abnormal discharge commonly associated with the disease was semen, or "seed.")

Gonorrhea is also known by several slang

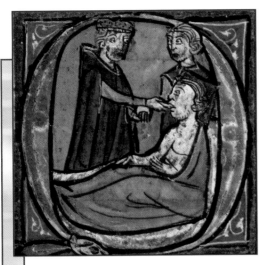

In this illustration from the thirteenth century, the ancient Greek physician Hippocrates treats a sick patient. Hippocrates is often considered the founder of modern medicine.

terms you may have heard before, such as "the drip" or "the clap." "The drip" refers to the symptom that Galen noticed, which is a pus-like discharge. Nobody knows quite where the nickname "the clap" came from, but there are a few reasonable guesses. An old French word, *clapier*, meant a brothel, or a house of prostitution, where cases of gonorrhea were probably widespread. The name may also have come from a woman named Mother Clap, who ran a brothel in London in the 1700s.

What Causes Gonorrhea

Now we know that gonorrhea is caused by a bacterium called *Neisseria gonorrhoeae*, which grows in warm, moist areas of the body such as the cervix, urethra, throat, rectum, or even the eyes. Bacteria are tiny, single-celled organisms that live all around us. Most bacteria are not detrimental, but some are. When these harmful bacteria get inside your system, they can grow and multiply, and cause health problems. Luckily, most of these are easily treated with antibiotics, so if a bacterial disease is caught and treated early, it won't have any long-term effects.

Gonorrhea spreads very easily: the bacteria that cause it can move from one person to another through contact with semen or vaginal fluid. The delicate tissues of the genitals, rectum, and throat are vulnerable to infection by these bacteria. Any type of unprotected sexual contact with an infected partner, whether vaginal, oral, or anal, is enough to transmit the disease. It can also be spread from an infected pregnant mother to her baby during childbirth. Gonorrhea is not spread through physical contact like hugging or kissing. This means that only people who are sexually active are at risk of contracting gonorrhea.

RATE OF INFECTION

In the United States, local STD prevention programs—which can include hospitals, doctors, or STD clinics—are required to report how many patients they treat each year for certain sexually transmitted diseases to the Centers for Disease Control and Prevention (CDC). The CDC is part of the Department of Health and Human Services, the main agency in the U.S. government for protecting the health and safety of American citizens. According to the CDC,

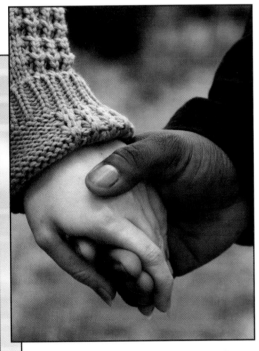

Unprotected sex—whether vaginal, oral, or anal—with an infected partner can spread gonorrhea. It is not possible to transmit or contract gonorrhea from casual physical contact, like hugging or holding hands.

more than 330,000 cases of gonorrhea were reported in the United States in 2004. However, because some cases are never diagnosed, and others just do not get reported, the number of cases reported is less than the actual number of cases occurring in the U.S. population. The CDC estimates that there may have been as many as 700,000 total cases of gonorrhea in 2004.

The CDC analyzes how many people in the United States are reported to have a particular disease in a particular year compared to the country's total population.

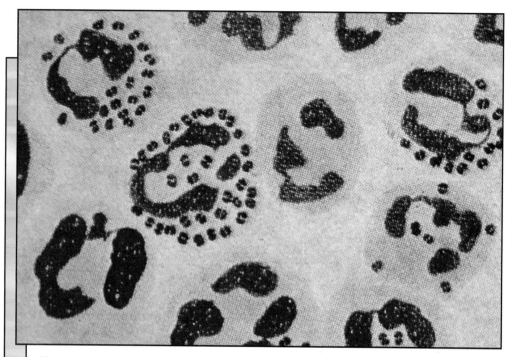

Neisseria gonorrhoeae bacteria, which cause gonorrhea, are visible through a microscope when a special staining technique is used.

Ten Facts About Gonorrhea

1. Gonorrhea has existed for thousands of years.

2. According to the CDC, the actual number of cases of gonorrhea in the United States is estimated to be more than twice the number of cases that are reported each year.

3. About half of the people infected with gonorrhea don't know it.

4. Currently, about 75 percent of all cases of gonorrhea are found in people between fifteen and twenty-nine years old.

5. In 2004, for the third straight year, females had a higher rate of gonorrhea infection than males.

6. Any sexually active person can be infected with gonorrhea. It can be transmitted during any kind of sexual contact: vaginal, oral, or anal.

7. In about 20 to 40 percent of gonorrhea cases, patients are also infected with chlamydia, another STD.

8. Having gonorrhea once doesn't mean you can't ever get it again, even if you have been treated and cured.

9. *Fluoroquinolone-Resistant N. gonorrhoeae* (QRNG), a drug-resistant form of gonorrhea, is spreading in Asia, the Pacific Islands (including Hawaii), California, and Great Britain.

10. If left untreated, long-term complications of gonorrhea such as pelvic inflammatory disease (PID) can develop.

For example, in 2004 the United States' population was about 290 million, so for that year, for every 100,000 people, 114 of them were reported to have a case of gonorrhea. This was the lowest rate of gonorrhea in recent years, showing that the rate of gonorrheal infection may be decreasing. Despite this good news, it is still very important to protect yourself. Gonorrhea is the second most commonly reported infectious disease. Chlamydia—another sexually transmitted bacterial infection—takes the number one spot. In 2004, there were 929,462 reported cases of chlamydia, almost two and a half times that of gonorrhea. The number of chlamydia cases continues to rise every year. The CDC can use statistics like these to show how levels of infection change over time, and to help decide the most effective ways to prevent the spread of STDs.

RISK FACTORS

There are several high-risk behaviors that can increase your chances of contracting an STD like gonorrhea. These include:

- Unprotected sex—that is, sex of any kind without the use of a condom or dental dam (a small sheet of latex that acts as a barrier between the vagina or anus and the mouth).
- Unprotected sexual activity at an early age. The rate of STD infection in younger age groups is increasing, so there is a growing chance that by having sex at a

Myths and Facts

MYTH: You can tell if someone has an STD just by looking at him or her.
FACT: Many STDs don't have obvious symptoms. Some people don't even know they're infected. Even someone who is attractive and dresses well can have an STD.

MYTH: My friends and I are too young to catch something like gonorrhea. It's something only older people have to worry about.
FACT: STDs are becoming much more common among young people. In the United States in 2004, the highest rates of infection for gonorrhea were found in fifteen- to nineteen-year-old women, and twenty- to twenty-four-year-old men. Approximately 75 percent of all cases of gonorrhea are found in people between fifteen and twenty-nine years of age.

MYTH: Engaging in only oral or anal sex, but not vaginal intercourse, is a safe way to prevent catching an STD.
FACT: Many STDs, including gonorrhea, can infect other areas of the body such as the throat, anus, or rectum. The delicate tissues of the rectum can actually make it more vulnerable to infection.

MYTH: You have to have multiple sexual partners to catch an STD.
FACT: Anyone who is sexually active is at risk of being infected, even if he or she has sex with only one person or has had sex just once. You can greatly reduce your risk of contracting an STD by always using latex condoms and dental dams, as appropriate, and by talking about your sexual history with your partner before you decide to become sexually active.

young age, you could be having sex with someone who has an STD.

- Unprotected sex with multiple partners. Each sexual partner has a chance of having an STD he or she can transmit to you. The greater number of partners you have, the greater number of chances you take.

• Drug injection, or having sex with a partner who injects drugs. Needles used for injecting drugs can also transmit disease, if they are shared with other people. In addition, drug use can lower inhibitions and cause you to do things you wouldn't normally do, like having sex without protection.

There are also certain populations that have a higher rate of gonorrhea and therefore have a higher risk of contracting the disease. According to the CDC, in 2004, 70 percent of the total number of gonorrhea cases reported occurred among African Americans. Rates of infection in African American men were twenty-six times higher than in Caucasian men, and fifteen times higher in African American women than in Caucasian women. Young people are also at a higher risk of contracting gonorrhea. About 75 percent of all cases reported in 2004 were found in people between fifteen and twenty-nine years old. There are even differences related to gender. In 2004, for the third straight year, females had a slightly higher rate of gonorrhea infection than males.

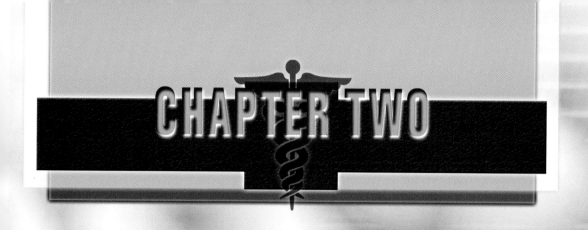

CHAPTER TWO

Symptoms of Gonorrhea

I f you become infected with the gonorrhea bacteria, it usually takes two to five days for symptoms to develop, but it can sometimes take up to thirty days. Symptoms are the signs and feelings your body uses to tell you that something is wrong. During that time, you can still transmit gonorrhea to other people, even though you don't have symptoms and may not know you have the disease.

About half the people infected with gonorrhea don't know it because they don't have any symptoms. Some people never develop symptoms. About 10 to 20 percent of males are asymptomatic, which means there are no obvious signs that they have been infected. Almost 50 percent of females who have gonorrhea are asymptomatic. This is one reason why the disease is easily spread. It is also why it is so important to be tested regularly for STDs once you're sexually active, even if you don't think you have a disease.

Symptoms can vary from patient to patient. Men and women may have some similar symptoms, but other symptoms may be different because of each gender's distinctive reproductive system. Symptoms can also differ depending on what part of the body is infected. For example, painful urination might be a symptom of a genital gonorrhea infection, but not if the bacteria have infected the throat as a result of unprotected oral sex.

SYMPTOMS IN MEN

Males have symptoms more often than females. Initial symptoms in men are usually noticeable enough that gonorrhea is detected before complications can occur. Symptoms in men most often include:

- An abnormal discharge, or liquid, from the penis. This discharge can range from a clear liquid to a thicker and sometimes bloody fluid.
- Pain or itching (may be severe) during urination.
- Frequent urination.
- Painful or swollen testicles or prostate gland.
- Fever of over 100 degrees Fahrenheit (37.8 degrees Celsius).
- If gonorrhea has been transmitted to the anus or rectum, symptoms can include anal itching, pain, bleeding, and abnormal discharge.
- If gonorrhea has been transmitted to the throat, a sore throat could be the only symptom.

SYMPTOMS IN WOMEN

Symptoms for women are often milder than for men. In fact, they can be so mild that they're often confused with a bladder infection. Symptoms most often include:

- Abnormal vaginal discharge.
- Irregular vaginal bleeding.
- Pain (may be severe) during urination.
- Frequent urination.
- Lower abdominal pain.
- Fever of over 100 degrees Fahrenheit (37.8 degrees Celsius).
- If gonorrhea has been transmitted to the anus or rectum, symptoms can include anal itching, pain, bleeding, and abnormal discharge.
- If gonorrhea has been transmitted to the throat, a sore throat could be the only symptom.

SYMPTOMS IN BABIES

If a pregnant mother passes gonorrhea to her infant during childbirth, the baby can also show symptoms. Conjunctivitis, or pinkeye, is very common in newborns of women with untreated gonorrhea. If not treated, it can lead to blindness. Doctors therefore usually treat all newborns with antibiotic eye drops soon after birth, just to be safe. A newborn baby might also have pneumonia, an inflammation of the lungs usually caused by infection from a bacterium or virus.

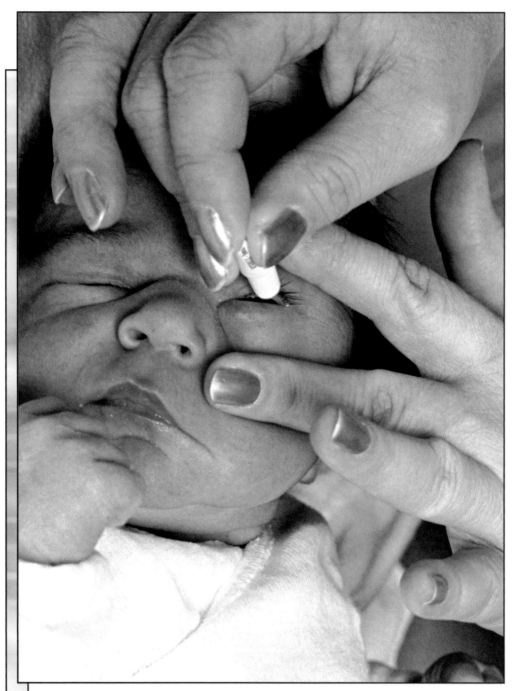

If a pregnant woman has gonorrhea, she can pass conjunctivitis to her baby during childbirth. Therefore, to be safe, most health-care professionals treat newborns with antibiotic eye drops shortly after birth.

COMPLICATIONS

If gonorrhea is detected and treated early, it has no long-term effects. However, serious problems can develop and affect the rest of your life if the infection is left untreated.

Gonorrhea becomes more serious if left untreated because the bacteria that cause it will continue to grow and can spread to other areas of the body. Most likely, the bacteria will spread to other parts of the reproductive system, but sometimes they can get into the bloodstream and spread throughout the body. For both men and women, this can cause widespread problems such as a rash or arthritis and joint pain. Bacterial growth can also create abscesses, which are hard-to-cure holes or pockets inside the body that fill with fluid. In addition, recent scientific studies provide strong evidence

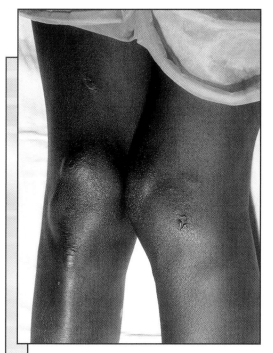

If gonorrhea is left untreated, the bacteria that cause the disease can enter the bloodstream and spread throughout the body. This can lead to complications including arthritic joints and skin lesions *(above)*.

that gonorrhea infection makes the body more susceptible, or vulnerable, to HIV (human immunodeficiency virus), the virus that causes AIDS (acquired immunodeficiency syndrome).

These long-term effects are why it's so important to see a doctor immediately at the first sign of symptoms, especially abdominal pain, abnormal discharge, a burning sensation during urination, and fever. Regular doctor visits for STD testing are also important since people with gonorrhea don't always have obvious symptoms. Your doctor can help find an infection so it can be treated right away, before complications occur.

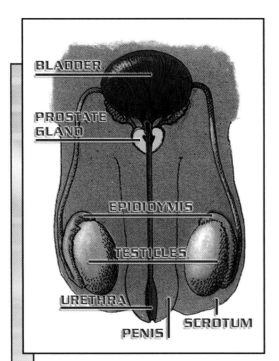

This diagram of the male reproductive system shows the scrotum, testicles, epididymis, urethra, and prostate, all of which risk damage from an untreated gonorrhea infection.

Complications in Men

Men are also at risk for gender-specific complications from gonorrhea. The most serious complication is a condition called epididymitis. This is a painful swelling of the scrotum, testicles, and the epididymis, a long, coiled tube that stores sperm. Epididymitis can cause sterility since damage to this tube can scar, interfering with the body's ability to store sperm or transport it during sexual intercourse. Other common complications include urethritis, a swelling and infection of the urethra (the tube that carries urine from the bladder), which can cause scarring of the urine canal. Prostatitis, a swelling and infection of the prostate gland, is another possible long-term complication.

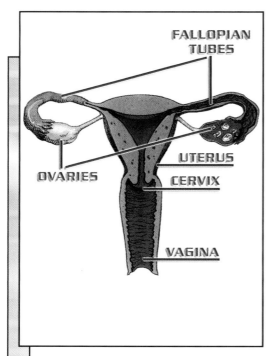

This diagram of the female reproductive system shows the uterus, fallopian tubes, and ovaries, which are vulnerable to pelvic inflammatory disease (PID) if gonorrhea is left untreated.

Complications in Women

For women, pelvic inflammatory disease (PID) is a very serious condition that can develop if gonorrhea is left untreated. PID is a swelling and infection of the female reproductive tract, including the uterus, fallopian tubes, and ovaries. Just like with the male reproductive tract, these tissues can scar, which can lead to chronic, or ongoing, pain. The scarring could block the fallopian tubes and cause sterility. If this happens, a fertilized egg may not be able to travel down the tube to the uterus, and might instead implant in the wall of the fallopian tube. This is called a tubal or ectopic pregnancy. An ectopic pregnancy is a very dangerous and possibly fatal condition.

Women may also experience chronic menstrual difficulties, postpartum endometriosis (inflammation of the lining of the uterus after pregnancy), and cystitis (inflammation of the bladder).

Pregnant women who have gonorrhea that has gone untreated are at further risk. They have a higher chance of having a miscarriage and going into premature labor.

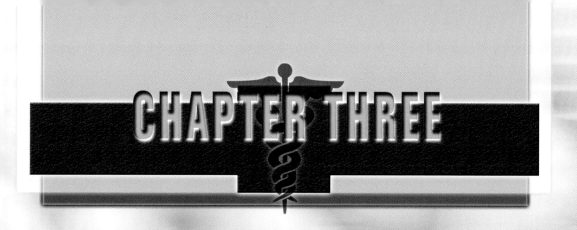

CHAPTER THREE

Detection and Treatment

I f you suspect that you might have gonorrhea or another STD, the first step in dealing with it is to see a doctor. You should have routine checkups and tests for STDs if you are sexually active regardless, since gonorrhea doesn't always have noticeable symptoms. Regular testing can result in the early detection of a disease. You can then deal with it before it causes long-term problems. Health-care professionals recommend being tested for STDs at least once a year if you're sexually active, and more frequently if you have new sexual partners during that time. If you find out that a person you had a sexual relationship with in the past has been diagnosed with an STD, get tested immediately to make sure you weren't infected.

SEEING A DOCTOR

If you notice symptoms, it's even more important to see a doctor and get tested. Remember that doctors are there to help you and make sure you're healthy. There's no reason to feel uncomfortable, embarrassed, or shy. He or

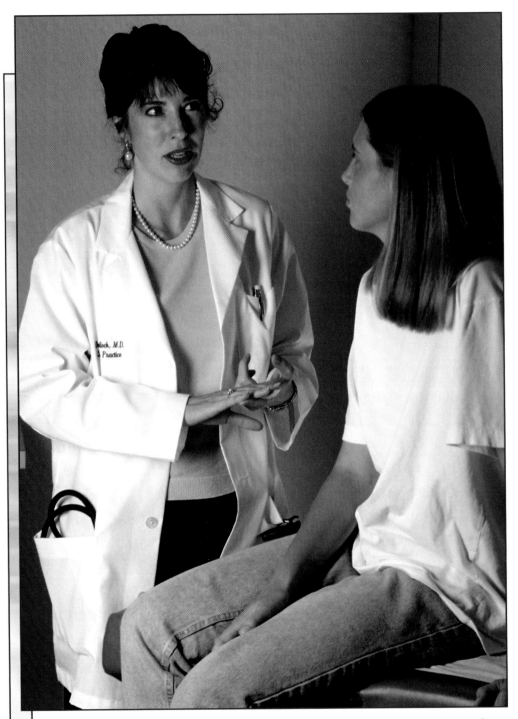

Seeing a doctor on a regular basis is an important part of staying healthy and protecting yourself from STDs. Listen carefully to your doctor's advice, and be sure to ask any questions you may have.

she may ask questions about your sexual history, your symptoms, whether you regularly use birth control and latex condoms, if you are sexually active, and if you engage in any high-risk sexual behaviors. Be sure to answer the doctor's questions honestly and share anything unusual. Your answers will help provide the fastest, most effective treatment.

You have the option of either visiting your regular doctor or going to any of a number of clinics. Other options may include local health departments and Planned Parenthood locations. Many cities sponsor public clinics that specialize in STD screening. The clinics are sometimes free, and some offer anonymous testing. Instead of names, patients are identified with numbers to protect their privacy. What testing site to visit is up to you. Ask yourself if you would feel more comfortable discussing these issues with a familiar doctor, or if you'd prefer to be tested somewhere else.

When you see a doctor, you should feel free to ask questions. Ask whatever you want to make yourself feel comfortable with the testing procedure and with any possible treatment.

DIAGNOSIS

In addition to asking about your medical history, a doctor will do several other things in order to diagnose you. He or she might conduct a pelvic or genital exam and look at any other affected area. In some cases you will be asked

1. What kind of tests should I have?

2. How could I have been infected?

3. Will I always have gonorrhea?

4. What treatments are available for the disease?

5. Once I'm cured, is it possible to get gonorrhea again?

6. How can I prevent this from happening again?

7. Could I have given gonorrhea to someone else?

8. Do my parents have to find out?

9. Will this disease hurt my chances of having children?

10. How can I talk to my partner about this?

for a urine sample, and other times a sample will be taken from either the inside of the penis or the vagina. There are several laboratory tests available to diagnose gonorrhea. These include:

- **Culture test:** A discharge sample is placed in a nutrient-rich environment and allowed to grow for forty-eight hours. After the bacteria in the sample have had a chance to multiply and be more easily seen, the sample is examined under a microscope.

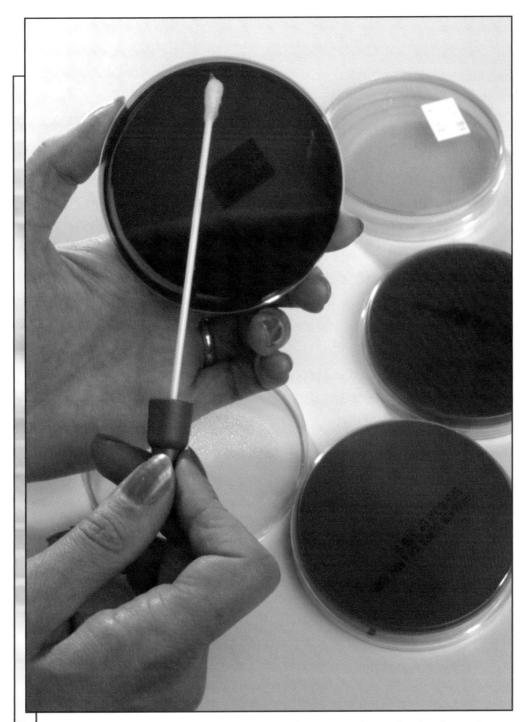

In a culture test, a cotton swab is used to take a vaginal sample. Any bacteria from the swab are transferred to a Petri dish. After allowing the bacteria time to multiply and grow, the sample is checked for the presence of *N. gonorrhoeae*.

A culture test can also be used to detect gonorrhea bacteria in the throat. This test is usually about 90 percent accurate for both men and women.

- **Gram stain test:** A sample of genital discharge is placed on a slide and stained with dye. The slide is then examined under a microscope to see if *N. gonorrhoeae*, the bacteria that cause gonorrhea, is present. This test works very well for men, but it is not effective for about half of women tested.
- **DNA test:** This test actually detects the DNA of gonorrhea bacteria and is the most accurate, although also the most expensive, of the available tests. DNA testing is becoming more common because it is the test most likely to accurately detect a gonorrhea infection.

TREATMENT

The only treatment for gonorrhea is antibiotics. Luckily, antibiotics are easily available and inexpensive, and a single dose is often enough to cure the infection completely. If complications have developed, however, treatment may be more involved. For example, surgery may be necessary to repair an abscess, but this is rare.

Antibiotics are a relatively new way to treat bacterial infections. It wasn't until the 1940s, during World War II, that field medics accidentally discovered that penicillin, an antibiotic, was highly effective in curing gonorrhea. Penicillin became the standard treatment for years.

Unfortunately, over time bacteria can become antibiotic-resistant. This means that a specific antibiotic no longer kills the bacteria that cause a particular disease. A different antibiotic must therefore be used to cure it.

Gonorrhea bacteria have become almost entirely resistant to penicillin and other common antibiotics, like tetracycline. Therefore, newly developed antibiotics are now being used. The most commonly prescribed antibiotics for gonorrhea are a type known as fluoro-quinolones and include ciprofloxacin, levofloxacin, and

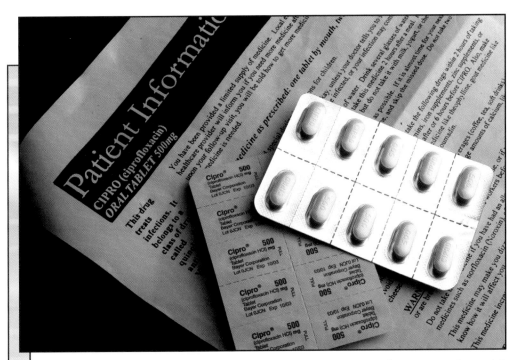

Ciprofloxacin, or Cipro, is one antibiotic a doctor may prescribe to treat a bacterial infection such as gonorrhea. There are several antibiotics a doctor can choose from to create the most effective treatment plan.

Treatment Myths

From ancient times to today, people have had some odd ideas about what would cure gonorrhea. For example, in Egypt, cold seawater was mixed with vinegar and forced into the penis at high pressure. Some people thought the disease could be cured by taking a lot of cold baths, or by wrapping the penis or vagina in wool. Even more remarkable, in Persia the treatment involved putting a live louse inside the urethra! Some people still mistakenly believe that gonorrhea can be cured by washing the infected area with a salt solution, or by drinking glass after glass of cranberry juice.

ofloxacin. These drugs can be used to cure several kinds of bacterial infections. Ciprofloxacin, for example, is the same antibiotic used to treat patients exposed to anthrax. In about 20 to 40 percent of gonorrhea cases, patients are also infected with chlamydia, another STD. Just to be safe, a doctor may decide to prescribe an additional antibiotic that treats chlamydia. This could include a course of antibiotics called azithromycin or doxycycline.

Continued research is necessary for gonorrhea treatment. These new antibiotics are already becoming less effective, so even newer and more powerful drugs are needed. Currently, there is a strain, or type, of gonorrhea known as *Fluoroquinolone-Resistant N. gonorrhoeae*, or QRNG. This strain is common in Asia, the Pacific Islands (including Hawaii), California, England, and Wales. QRNG must be treated with different, stronger antibiotics such as ceftriaxone or cefixime. As well as trying to make new antibiotics, researchers examine how gonorrhea becomes resistant to existing antibiotics. These studies lead to faster, more effective treatments for the disease.

The antibiotics can usually be administered in a single dose, by pill or injection, depending on the particular drug. If the bacteria have spread, a longer course of antibiotics may be necessary. Be sure to take all of the medication, for the entire specified time period, even if the symptoms have disappeared. Otherwise, the infection may not be entirely gone, and could come back stronger

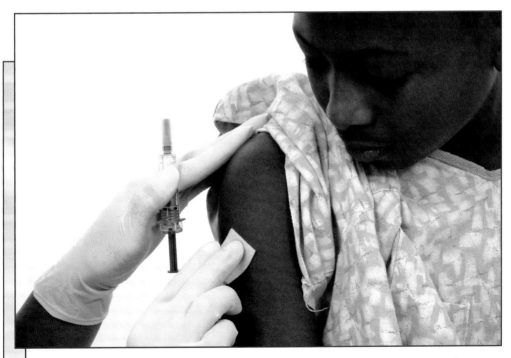

Depending on the treatment a doctor prescribes, medication to cure gonorrhea could involve an injection of antibiotics instead of pills or tablets.

than ever and resistant to the antibiotics. Wait until treatment is complete and successful before engaging in sexual activity of any kind. Otherwise, you risk passing the disease to others.

AFTER THE DIAGNOSIS

Doctors are usually required by law to report an STD diagnosis to the local health department. This information is used for statistical purposes and can help the health department develop new strategies for dealing with and eliminating STDs. Doctors are not required by law to inform parents about their teenager's diagnosis or treatment, although several states allow them to do so, if they think it is in the teen's best interests. If you are concerned about this, ask your doctor.

After you have been diagnosed and begun treatment, it is very important for your past and present sexual partners to be tested. You may have transmitted the disease to them, just as easily as they might have given it to you. If necessary, they will also need to be treated. Remember, you must wait until they have finished treatment before you can have sexual contact again, or else you risk re-infection. Unlike diseases such as chicken pox, having gonorrhea once doesn't mean you can't get it again. Every time you are exposed, you are just as likely to get it, and each time carries the same risks and requires antibiotics. If you are too embarrassed to tell your current or previous partners, some health care professionals will gather

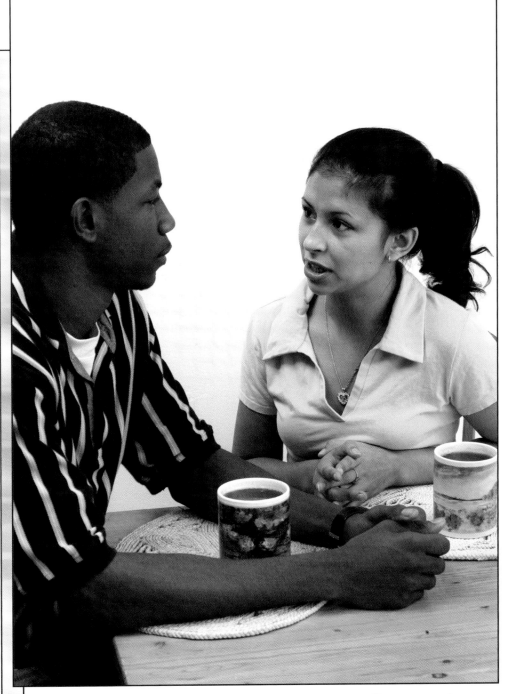

If you have been diagnosed with an STD, it is important to tell any past and present sexual partners. If someone with whom you have had a sexual relationship tells you he or she has been diagnosed with an STD, you should get tested, too.

contact information and call them for you. It is very important that your partners be tested.

It is also crucial to figure out what you did to become infected. Did you take part in high-risk activity? Did you use a latex condom or dental dam every time you engaged in sexual activity? What changes can you make to prevent another infection?

Think about what questions to ask future sexual partners before you have sex. Asking these questions can help you to decide what you want and don't want to do with them. Making well-informed choices is one of the safest, surest ways you have to protect yourself from contracting an STD.

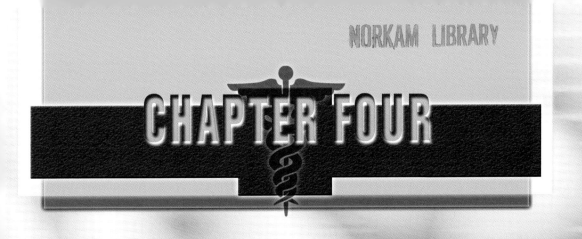

CHAPTER FOUR

Prevention

G onorrhea is one of the oldest, most widespread sexually transmitted diseases in the world; it's not always obvious that a sexual partner has the disease; and it's easy to contract. How, then, can you protect yourself from gonorrhea? Is it inevitable that you're going to become infected? Thankfully, no. Some behaviors are riskier than others. There are steps you can take, however, to greatly reduce your risk of becoming infected with gonorrhea and many other STDs. All it takes is some forethought.

SEXUAL ACTIVITY

Sexual activity puts you at risk of contracting a disease like gonorrhea. If you have decided to become sexually active and you and your partner are not careful to take measures to protect yourselves, pregnancy and STDs are possibilities that come with the territory. These consequences can be severe and life-changing, so it is important that you are making the right choices for you.

You might become sexually active for a number of reasons. You might want to show someone how much you care about him or her. Often, peer pressure is a factor. You might have sex with your partner because he or she wants you to, or because you think you have to. Sometimes, a partner who wants to start a sexual relationship can be very insistent and try to convince you to do something you don't really want to do. He or she may try to make you feel guilty for not having sex. You might even be worried that he or she will break up with you if you don't have sex. If this happens, remember that everyone has the right to control his or her own body. A partner who cares about you will understand your decision. If someone does get angry with you, or even breaks up with you because you don't have sex, it is a poor reflection of his or her character, not yours. You might feel embarrassed or hurt in such a situation, but in the long run, that's much easier to deal with than a serious problem like an STD.

SEX AND THE MEDIA

The media's portrayal of sexual behavior can influence your decision as well. Often, on television and in movies, characters are seen engaging in sexual activity without any real-life consequences. This attitude is unrealistic and can even be dangerous. It is important to remember that these characters are not real, so they don't have to be concerned with the many issues you will need to think about. A February 2002 article in the *Journal of Sex Research*

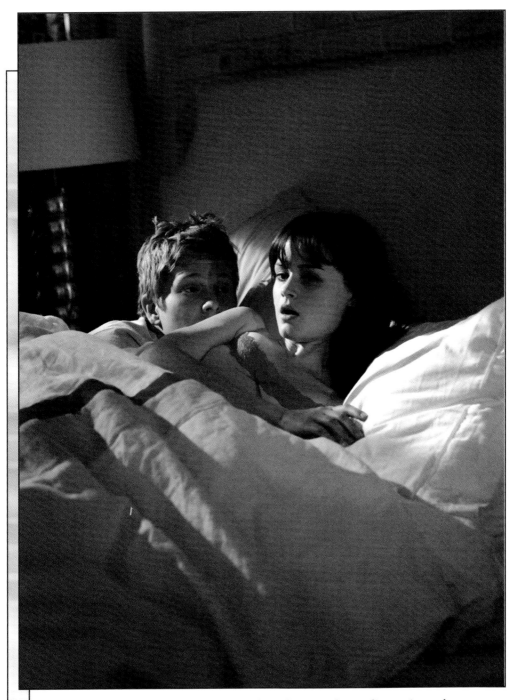

Characters in movies or on TV often don't have realistic discussions about or attitudes toward sexual activity. In the above image from the WB's *The Gilmore Girls*, Rory Gilmore (Alex Bledel) wakes up with her boyfriend Logan Huntzberger (Matt Czuchry).

describes the media's influence on sexuality and its depiction of "the three C's": Commitment, Contraceptives, and Consequences. People having sex on the screen are often shown as not being committed to each other: either they are strangers, have just met, or don't have a relationship after their sexual encounter. Use of contraceptives (birth control) is also rarely addressed: only about one in ten television programs containing sexual content discuss the need to use birth control or protection. In addition, television and movies almost never discuss the possible unwanted consequences of sex such as pregnancy or catching an STD.

The essential thing to remember is that these movies and TV shows are not taking place in the real world. They don't show how actual relationships work, and therefore are not necessarily a good model for how you should behave. An honest discussion is the best way for you to decide if you're ready—mentally and emotionally—to take on the responsibilities of being sexually active.

ABSTINENCE

If you decide you're not ready to be sexually active, the alternative is abstinence. "Abstinence" means refraining from sexual activity of any kind. It is the only way to be 100 percent sure to avoid the risk of pregnancy or sexually transmitted infection.

If you are abstinent, you don't have any kind of sexual intercourse, including oral sex or anal sex, which are also ways to contract an STD. Some STDs, such as genital herpes or genital warts, can even be spread by skin-to-skin contact with an infected area. Physical intimacy certainly does not have to be avoided altogether, however. Hugging, touching, massaging of non-genital areas, kissing, and rubbing or petting each other with your clothes on are all safe activities.

If you decide to be abstinent, it is best to determine boundaries with your partner ahead of time. Clearly define what these boundaries are, and make sure that you and

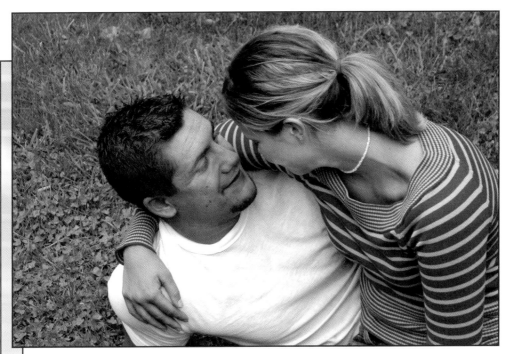

A couple can do lots of things to be physically close that don't involve having sex. Hugging, touching, and kissing are all activities that keep you safe from STDs, but also let you show affection to your partner.

your partner both understand them. It might be difficult to stick to these choices in the heat of the moment, but if you decide on them beforehand, you can be sure that they're the right decisions for you.

SAFER SEX

If, after careful consideration and discussion, you decide to become sexually active, it is crucial to protect yourself and your partner by practicing safe sex, every single time you have sex. Safe sex is not 100 percent safe.

The following tips, however, are important to follow for safer sex:

- Use a latex condom and dental dam (a small sheet of latex that acts as a barrier between the vagina or anus and the mouth). They are the best ways to reduce your risk of STD transmission. It might feel embarrassing to buy condoms, but it is one of the most grown-up and responsible things you can do to take care of yourself and your partner. Many local health departments and Planned Parenthood locations give away condoms.
- Become familiar with the different types of condoms available. There are both male and female condoms, and condoms made of different materials. Some of these, such as latex condoms, prevent pregnancy as well as the spread of STDs. If you are allergic to latex, you can use polyurethane condoms, which are

made from a type of plastic. Natural, or lambskin, condoms are effective barriers to pregnancy, but not to many of the organisms that can cause a STDs, so it's very important to use latex or polyurethane.

- Store condoms in a cool, dry place (not in a pocket, wallet, or glove compartment).
- Be sure to use a fresh, unbroken condom. Never re-use a condom!
- Open the package carefully (don't use your teeth or scissors), and check the expiration date on the wrapper.

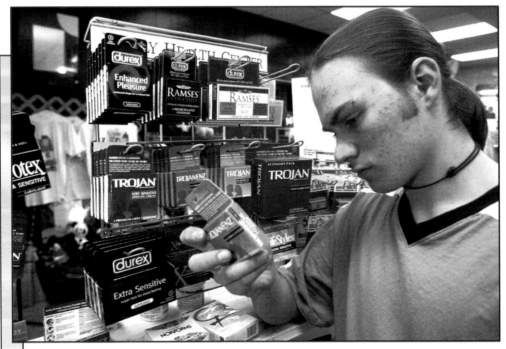

There is no such thing as 100 percent safe sex. If you are sexually active, it is important to use latex condoms, which help prevent STDs as well as pregnancy.

- Know how to use contraceptives properly. Put on a condom after the penis is erect, but before there is any genital contact.
- Ejaculation doesn't need to occur for transmission of a disease. After ejaculation, immediately remove the condom and dispose of it properly to avoid spilling any semen that has collected.
- Birth control pills are only effective against pregnancy, not STDs. Condoms must be used to prevent the transmission of STDs.
- Use regularly lubricated condoms instead of condoms lubricated with spermicide. Condoms lubricated with spermicide are not more effective, and spermicide can cause vaginal irritation, which makes it more likely for STDs to be transmitted.
- Condoms are very good at preventing pregnancy and the spread of infection, but they are not 100 percent effective.

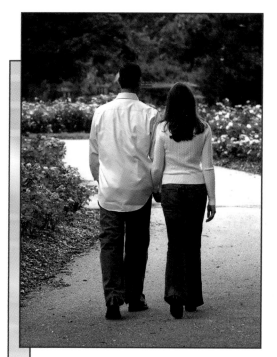

Communication in a relationship is important. Before engaging in sexual activity with your partner, take time to discuss your past sexual histories.

The only absolutely certain way to be safe is to practice abstinence.

THE IMPORTANCE OF COMMUNICATION

In addition to physical protection such as condoms, communicating with your partner is important. You might feel embarrassed to discuss some of these issues, but it's an excellent idea to be sure that you both understand what you're doing. Discussion can minimize pressure, confusion, and arguments because you will know the other's boundaries. If you and your partner decide to have sex, discuss your sexual histories beforehand. Talk about any high-risk behaviors, and try to answer questions honestly. Making an appointment to be screened for sexually transmitted diseases together may be helpful. Identify birth control options and what you each can do to limit the spread of STDs.

Good communication doesn't end there. Discuss any health issues or problems that arise with your partner and your doctor. Also, be aware of what your bodies are telling you. If you or your partner has any unusual symptoms, get them checked out. If you ever feel uncomfortable with any sexual activities, talk about your feelings. Being sexually active is one of the closest relationships you can have with another person. It is fine to feel embarrassed or shy with your partner, but try to communicate your needs, wants, and concerns.

The more you talk about issues, the closer you will become and the happier you both will be.

MULTIPLE PARTNERS VS. MONOGAMY

Having sex with multiple people in a short period of time may increase your risk of contracting a sexually transmitted disease. The more partners you have, the more chances you take of being exposed to an STD. Before and after each sexual relationship, you should be screened for STDs.

A mutually monogamous relationship means that you and your partner have both agreed that you will have sex with each other, and only each other. If you have a committed sexual relationship, once you've both been tested and cleared of any disease, you should have no risk of catching an STD from each other. (To avoid pregnancy, birth control should remain an important part of your sexual activity.) Unfortunately, since not everyone is honest when it comes to sex, an agreement of monogamy is not a guarantee. You should therefore both continue to be screened for STDs. And remember, if you enter a relationship with a new partner, you need to have the same discussions and take the same precautions that you did with your previous partner.

SUBSTANCE USE AND SEXUAL ACTIVITY

Using controlled substances like alcohol or drugs can be dangerous, not just because of what they do to your body, but also how they affect your judgment. Under the influence of drugs or alcohol, carefully considered decisions may be completely forgotten, and you may do things that you normally would not consider.

Alcohol and drugs can seriously impair your ability to make good decisions. Staying sober helps make sure that the decisions you make with your partner are decisions you can stick to. If you use alcohol or drugs, you are much more likely to engage in other risky behaviors, like having sex with someone with whom you have not discussed the consequences, or having unprotected sex. Just like with sexual activity, peer pressure or the media can glamorize substance abuse. Remember, you have the right to decide what to do with your body, and that includes what substances you put into it.

All of these methods are good ways to minimize your chances of catching gonorrhea or other sexually transmitted diseases. It is important to know, however, that abstinence is the only surefire way to avoid the risk entirely.

CHAPTER FIVE

Coping with the Disease

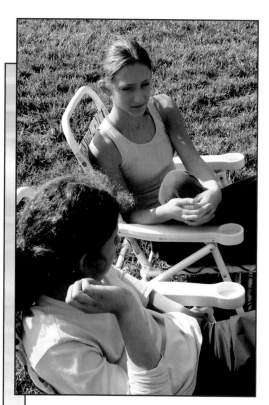

The emotional consequences of a disease may be just as difficult to deal with as the physical ones. Family and friends can be a great source of support.

I f you discover that you have contracted gonorrhea, try to stay calm. Think about the complications that can result if the disease is left untreated, and talk to a doctor right away. Let your partner know that there's a problem, and stop all sexual contact until you're absolutely certain that you have been completely cured. In addition to looking out for your own health, you have a responsibility to prevent spreading the disease to others.

Jon's Story

Jon is a sophomore in high school. Last year, he was really excited to attend a new school and meet all of the other new students. He was a little shy at first, until a girl named Amanda from his biology class asked him to join her and her friends at their lunch table.

Jon spent a lot of time hanging out at lunch and after school with his new group of friends, especially Amanda. She was athletic, attractive, and smart; Jon had a big crush on her. He wanted to ask her out, but he felt too nervous when she was around and didn't really know what to say. Amanda solved the problem by kissing Jon while they were doing math homework one afternoon. It may not have made Jon feel any less nervous around her, but at least he knew that the feeling was mutual.

They spent a lot of time together, and slowly they became more physical with each other. Eventually, they talked a few times about having sex, usually when they had been making out for a while. At first Amanda talked Jon out of it. After they had been going out for a number of months, however, she told Jon that she had a surprise for him. Her parents were going out of town for the weekend, and she invited him to spend the night. Jon didn't have any condoms, but Amanda was already taking birth control pills, and she said that having sex would be completely safe.

After that weekend, they continued to have sex. Jon was too embarrassed to buy condoms, and he didn't want to talk about buying them with Amanda either. Jon was a little worried, but he figured that Amanda knew what she was talking about. A few weeks after they started sleeping together, however, Jon started to feel severe pain when he urinated. He figured he must have a bladder infection. He had heard stories that cranberry juice was supposed to cure bladder infections, so he drank a lot of it, hoping the symptoms would go away. The juice had little effect other than to make him sick of cranberry juice. He started avoiding Amanda because he was afraid she would notice that there was something wrong with him. He was also too embarrassed to talk to his parents.

The pain got worse over the next few days, and finally Jon couldn't take it anymore. He told his mom he was feeling sick and thought he might have strep throat, but when he went to the doctor, Jon told him about his real symptoms. The doctor asked him several questions, including whether he was sexually active. Jon was worried that the doctor

continued on following page

continued from previous page

would be angry or get him in trouble with his parents if he told him. He answered the doctor's questions honestly, though, and the doctor was very friendly and professional. Jon's doctor told him about the tests that he was going to run and that he would contact Jon in a few days with the results.

When the tests showed that Jon had gonorrhea, he was shocked. He had always thought that STDs happened only to people who have sex with many different people or who use drugs. His doctor told him how STDs can be contracted and explained that Jon had to talk to Amanda about getting tested, too. The doctor gave him a few suggestions about how he could bring up the conversation and told him to stay calm. Since Jon didn't want his parents to know he had gonorrhea, he paid for the antibiotics he needed. Then he went to talk to Amanda.

Although Jon knew that Amanda was the only person he had ever had sex with, and therefore he must have contracted gonorrhea from her, he was still worried about telling her. Even though he knew it didn't make sense, he was concerned that she was going to be mad at him. He decided to tell her that he had just gone to the doctor and that he had to take antibiotics. When Amanda asked Jon what was wrong, he gathered his courage and asked Amanda if she had slept with other people before him. She didn't want to talk about it until Jon let her know how important it was to him. She told him that she had had a boyfriend the year before she met Jon, and they had had sex. Jon calmly discussed gonorrhea the way the doctor told him. He also explained how Amanda might be unaware she even had the disease. He stressed that she needed to be tested—and so would her old boyfriend.

For a while, Jon was angry that Amanda had given him gonorrhea, but he gradually realized it was partly his fault, too. After talking with his doctor, Jon knew that he and Amanda should have discussed their past sexual histories before they started having sex with each other. They also should have used condoms every time. Happily, Jon and Amanda have been treated and cured, and they are both disease-free. They are still dating, and Jon feels a lot closer to Amanda now, too. Once you're brave enough to talk about STDs and birth control with someone, you can really talk to them about anything!

As well as possible physical consequences, sexual activity has possible emotional consequences. There are ways to cope if you're diagnosed with an STD, however. There are also ways you can help if a friend or family member contracts a sexually transmitted disease.

EMOTIONS AND SEXUAL ACTIVITY

As Jon's story on the previous pages demonstrates, becoming sexually active can make you feel a lot of different things. It might be exciting as you learn to deal with the responsibilities that come with sexual activity. It may make you feel vulnerable, because a sexual relationship is brand new and requires you to be open to another person in a way that you're not with anybody else. You might feel nervous, or even a little scared. You might have to feel brave to overcome some embarrassment and discuss these topics with someone.

Similarly, there are a lot of possible emotions if you contract an STD. You might feel ashamed or embarrassed or alone. You might be afraid of what could happen if your friends or family find out. You might be worried about how your partner will react when you say that he or she will need to be tested for an STD. You might be angry with your partner for transmitting a disease to you. You could even be scared of having sex ever again.

If someone you know has an STD and shares the information with you, think about how you'd want them to react if the situation was reversed. He or she might be feeling scared, and the best thing you can do is be supportive. Don't laugh or get angry. Help your friend deal with it effectively. He or she will really appreciate your support.

One of the best ways to deal with all of these feelings is to get more information. The knowledge will help you with future decisions.

POSITIVE STEPS

Being diagnosed with a sexually transmitted disease provides a very good opportunity to make positive changes in your life. No matter what you have done in the past, it is never too late to improve how you deal with important issues like your relationships, your sexual activity, and your health.

Examples of positive steps may include a resolution to practice safe sex every time you have sex, or a determination to have an in-depth conversation with your partner about his or her sexual history. A positive step can also be a decision to improve your general health by eating better, exercising, or getting enough sleep.

Acting in such a constructive fashion will counter any negative emotions you might be experiencing as a result of your diagnosis. As you move forward by putting these choices into practice, not only will you start to feel better physically, you will feel better emotionally, too.

RESOURCES AND PEOPLE WHO CAN HELP

There are a lot of people and places you can go to for help. The most important could be your family or friends. You might be worried about getting in trouble if you tell your parents or family members, but they'll probably be very glad you can be so honest and open with them. Talk about your situation calmly, and ask them for advice on what you can do to be healthy and make well-informed decisions.

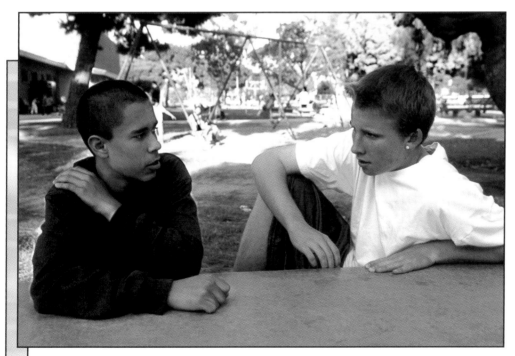

Someone you know may need help coping with an STD diagnosis. Listen to your friend and be honest and supportive.

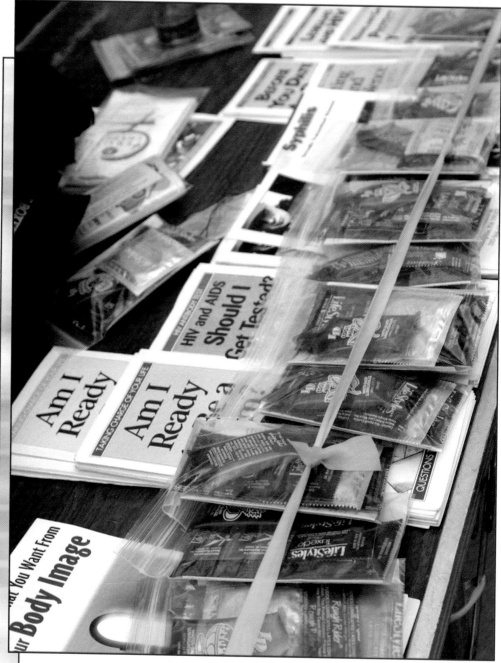

Support groups, Web sites, telephone hotlines, and even pamphlets from your doctor or a local clinic are all good resources for information and help. Being well informed is one of the best ways to protect yourself from a sexually transmitted disease.

Friends are also a great source of support. They can provide advice or just a shoulder to lean on. Your doctor or another health-care professional will be happy to give you information on how to make healthy choices. You might like to talk to a religious leader in your life, too, like a priest, minister, or rabbi. If you don't feel comfortable asking any of these people, there are lots of support groups, Web sites, and telephone hotlines that will provide more information. There are lists of references at the end of this book that can help.

When it comes to gonorrhea or any other sexually transmitted disease, the smartest thing you can do is be informed. Thinking about the issues raised in this book and talking about them with your family and friends will help make sure that you know what's best for you. It's important to learn how to be responsible, be healthy, make good choices, and protect yourself.

GLOSSARY

abstinence Refraining from sexual activity of any kind, whether oral, vaginal, or anal. Also called celibacy.

antibiotic-resistant No longer responding to a specific antibiotic.

antibiotics Medicine used to cure bacterial infections, including gonorrhea.

bacteria Microscopic organisms that can cause disease.

condom A thin protective barrier, usually made of latex, that is worn either over the penis or inside the vagina during sexual intercourse.

conjunctivitis Inflammation and irritation of the eye. Also called pinkeye.

contraceptives Methods of birth control.

culture test A test for gonorrhea that allows a sample to grow in a nutrient-rich environment to locate the gonorrhea bacteria.

dental dam A small sheet of latex that acts as a barrier between the vagina or anus and the mouth.

discharge The flow of pus, mucus, or other liquid from infected tissue.

DNA test A test for gonorrhea that looks for the genetic material of the gonorrhea bacteria.

epididymitis The painful swelling of the scrotum and testicles, and of a long, coiled tube called the epididymis that stores sperm. Can lead to infertility.

gram stain test A test for gonorrhea that uses dye to locate the gonorrhea bacteria.

infectious Able to spread an infection to other people.

infertile Unable to have children.

Neisseria gonorrhoeae The bacteria that causes gonorrhea.

pelvic inflammatory disease (PID) The painful swelling of the uterus, fallopian tubes, or ovaries. Can lead to infertility.

pneumonia A disease of the lungs characterized by inflammation of lung tissue, fever, cough, and difficulty breathing.

postpartum The period after giving birth.

sexually transmitted disease (STD) A disease passed from person to person through sexual contact. Also called a sexually transmitted infection (STI).

FOR MORE INFORMATION

Advocates for Youth
2000 M Street NW, Suite 750
Washington, DC 20036
(202) 419-3420
Web site: http://www.advocatesforyouth.org
Creates programs and advocates for policies that help
young people make informed, responsible decisions about
reproductive and sexual health. Advocates for Youth also
provides information, training, and assistance to organiza-
tions, policy makers, youth activists, and the media.

American Social Health Association (ASHA)
P.O. Box 13827
Research Triangle Park, NC 27709-3827
(919) 361-8400
STI Resource Center Hotline: (800) 227-8922
Web site: http://www.ashastd.org
ASHA provides information about STDs, tips for reducing
risk, and ways to talk with health care providers and
partners. Also a good source for referrals and help groups.

Canadian Federation for Sexual Health (CFSH)
1 Nicholas Street, Suite 430

Ottawa, ON K1N 7B7
Canada
(613) 241-4474
Web site: http://www.ppfc.ca
An organization that provides free education, services, information, and counseling for issues related to sexual health, birth control, and STDs.

Centers for Disease Control and Prevention (CDC)
1600 Clifton Road
Atlanta, GA 30333
(404) 639-3311
STD Hotline: (800) 232-4636
Web site: http://www.cdc.gov/std
The CDC offers information on STDs, including how to prevent them. Its STD hotline provides referrals to clinics and other services.

Health Canada: Sexual Health and Promotion
Address Locator 0900C2
Ottawa, ON K1A 0K9
Canada
(866) 225-0709
Web site: http://www.hc-sc.gc.ca/hl-vs/sex/index_e.html
Health Canada promotes healthy sexuality by making information—based on current scientific research—readily available through publications, promotional resources, links, policies, and guidelines.

Planned Parenthood Federation of America
810 Seventh Avenue
New York, NY 10019
(800) 230-PLAN
Web site: http://www.plannedparenthood.org
Planned Parenthood provides sexual and reproductive
health care and education. Its Web site offers information
about birth control, STDs, and referrals to local clinics.

Sexuality Information and Education Council of the
    United States (SIECUS)
130 West 42nd Street, Suite 350
New York, NY 10036-7802
(212) 819-9770
Web site: http://www.siecus.org
SIECUS promotes comprehensive education about sexuality,
STDs, and responsible sexual choices.

WEB SITES

Due to the changing nature of Internet links, the Rosen
Publishing Group, Inc., has developed an online list of
Web sites related to the subject of this book. This site is
updated regularly. Please use this link to access the list:

http://www.rosenlinks.com/lsh/gono

FOR FURTHER READING

Basso, Michael J. *The Underground Guide to Teenage Sexuality*, 2nd ed. Minneapolis, MN: Fairview Press, 2003.

Bell, Ruth. *Changing Bodies, Changing Lives: A Book for Teens on Sex and Relationships*, 3rd ed. New York, NY: Three Rivers Press, 1998.

Harris, Robie H. *It's Perfectly Normal: Changing Bodies, Growing Up, Sex, and Sexual Health*. Cambridge, MA: Candlewick Press, 2004.

Hatchell, Deborah. *What Smart Teenagers Know . . . About Dating, Relationships, and Sex*. Santa Barbara, CA: Piper Books, 2003.

McCoy, Kathy. *The Teenage Body Book*. New York, NY: Perigee Books, 1999.

Solin, Sabrina, and Paula Elbirt. *Seventeen Guide to Sex and Your Body*. New York, NY: Aladdin Books, 1996.

Stanley, Deborah A., ed. *Sexual Health Information for Teens: Health Tips about Sexual Development, Human Reproduction, and Sexually Transmitted Diseases*. Detroit, MI: Omnigraphics, 2003.

Westheimer, Ruth. *Dr. Ruth Talks to Kids: Where You Came From, How Your Body Changes, and What Sex Is All About*. New York, NY: Aladdin Books, 1998.

BIBLIOGRAPHY

Brown, Jane D. "Mass Media Influences on Sexuality."
    Journal of Sex Research, February 2002.

Centers for Disease Control and Prevention (CDC).
    "Gonorrhea—CDC Fact Sheet." May 2004. Retrieved
    January 30, 2006 (http://www.cdc.gov/std/
    Gonorrhea/STDFact-gonorrhea.htm).

Guttmacher Institute. "State Policies in Brief: Minors'
    Access to STD Services." Retrieved February 21, 2006
    (http://www.guttmacher.org/statecenter/spibs/
    spib_MASS.pdf).

Hinton, Anna. "Sexually Transmitted Infections." Retrieved
    January 30, 2006 (http://www.brookes.ac.uk/student/
    services/health/sti.html).

Hunter, Miranda, and William Hunter. *Staying Safe?: A Teen's
    Guide to Sexually Transmitted Diseases*. Broomall, PA:
    Mason Crest Publishers, 2005.

Kolesnikow, Tassia. *Sexually Transmitted Diseases*.
    Farmington Hills, MI: Lucent Books, 2004.

National Institute of Allergy and Infectious Diseases
    (NIAID). "Gonorrhea." October 2004. Retrieved
    January 30, 2006 (http://www.niaid.nih.gov/
    factsheets/stdgon.htm).

WebMD. "Gonorrhea." May 2005. Retrieved January 30, 2006 (http://www.webmd.com/hw/std/aa33140.asp).

Yancey, Diane. *STDs: What You Don't Know Can Hurt You.* Brookfield, CT: Twenty-First Century Books, 2002.

INDEX

ABOUT THE AUTHOR

Christopher Michaud has a degree in molecular, cellular, and developmental biology from the University of Colorado at Boulder. He lives in New York City.

PHOTO CREDITS

Cover, p. 4 © www.istockphoto.com/ericsphotography; cover, pp. 1, 4 (silhouette) © www.istockphoto.com/jamesbenet; p. 1 (inset) CDC/Joe Miller; p. 5 Still Picture Records, National Archives and Records Administration; p. 7 akg-images/British Library; p. 9 © www.istockphoto.com/Chrissie Sheperd; p. 10 CDC; p. 18 © SIU/Peter Arnold, Inc.; p. 19 CDC/Emory University, Dr. Thomas F. Sellers; pp. 20, 21 Guilano Fornari Sergio © Dorling Kindersley; p. 24 © Will & Deni McIntyre/Photo Researchers, Inc.; p. 27 © Jim Varney/Photo Researchers, Inc.; p. 29 © Eliot J. Schechter/Getty Images; p. 31 © www.istockphoto.com; p. 33 © Colin Young-Wolff/PhotoEdit, Inc.; p. 35 © Warner Bros./Courtesy Everett Collection; p. 37 © Sean O'Brien/Custom Medical Stock Photo; p. 39 © Peter Bryon/PhotoEdit, Inc.; p. 40 © www.istockphoto.com/Brad Thompson; p. 45 © Mary Kate Denny/PhotoEdit, Inc.; p. 51 © www.istockphoto.com/Gallina Barskaya; p. 52 © Jeff Fusco/Getty Images; back cover (top to bottom) CDC/Dr. E. Arum, Dr. N. Jacobs, CDC/Dr. Edwin P. Ewing Jr., CDC/Joe Miller, CDC/Joe Miller, CDC/Dr. Edwin P. Ewing Jr., CDC.

Designer: Nelson Sá; **Editor:** Elizabeth Gavril
Photo Researcher: Nicole DiMella